PEER REVIEW & QUALITY COMMITTEE

Essentials Handbook

Richard A. Sheff, MD
Robert J. Marder, MD

Peer Review & Quality Committee Essentials Handbook is published by HCPro, Inc.

Copyright © 2012 HCPro, Inc.

ISBN: 978-1-60146-944-1

HCPro, Inc., provides information resources for the healthcare industry.

HCPro, Inc., is not affiliated in any way with The Joint Commission, which owns the JCAHO and Joint Commission trademarks.

Richard A. Sheff, MD, Author

Robert J. Marder, MD, Author

Katrina Gravel, Editorial Assistant

Elizabeth Jones, Editor

Erin Callahan, Associate Editorial Director

Mike Mirabello, Graphic Artist

Matt Sharpe, Production Supervisor

Shane Katz, Art Director

Jean St. Pierre, Senior Director of Operations

Advice given is general. Readers should consult professional counsel for specific legal, ethical, or clinical questions.

Arrangements can be made for quantity discounts. For more information, contact:

HCPro, Inc.

75 Sylvan Street, Suite A-101

Danvers, MA 01923

Telephone: 800-650-6787 or 781-639-1872

Fax: 800-639-8511

Email: *customerservice@hcpro.com*

Visit HCPro online at: *www.hcpro.com*
and *www.hcmarketplace.com*

Contents

Chapter 6: Ethical and Legal Issues: Discoverability, Conflict of Interest, and Confidentiality 69

Chapter 7: Efficient Peer Review Meetings. 77

     PEER REVIEW & QUALITY COMMITTEE ESSENTIALS HANDBOOK

Figure List

About the Authors

Richard A. Sheff, MD

Richard A. Sheff, MD, is principal and chief medical officer with The Greeley Company, a division of HCPro, Inc., in Danvers, Mass. He brings more than 25 years of healthcare management and leadership experience to his work with physicians, hospitals, and healthcare systems across the country. With his distinctive combination of medical, healthcare, and management acumen, Dr. Sheff develops tailored solutions for the unique needs of physicians and hospitals. He consults, authors, and presents on a wide range of healthcare management and leadership issues, including governance, physician–hospital alignment, medical staff leadership development, emergency department call, peer review, hospital performance improvement, disruptive physician management, conflict resolution, physician employment and contracting, healthcare systems, service line management, hospitalist program optimization, patient safety and error reduction, credentialing, strategic planning, regulatory compliance, and helping physicians rediscover the joy of medicine.

Robert J. Marder, MD

Robert J. Marder, MD, is an advisory consultant and director of medical staff services with The Greeley Company, a division of HCPro, Inc., in Danvers, Mass. He brings more than 25 years of healthcare leadership and management experience to his work with physicians, hospitals, and healthcare organizations across the country. Dr. Marder's many roles in senior hospital medical administration and operations management in academic and community hospital settings make him uniquely qualified to assist physicians and hospitals in developing solutions for complex medical staff and hospital performance issues. He consults, authors, and presents on a wide range of healthcare leadership issues, including effective and efficient peer review, physician performance measurement and improvement, hospital quality measurement systems and performance improvement, patient safety/error reduction, and utilization management.

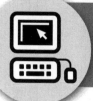

DOWNLOAD YOUR MATERIALS NOW

This handbook includes a customizable presentation that organizations can use to train physician leaders. The presentation complements the information provided in this handbook and can be downloaded at the following link:

www.hcpro.com/downloads/10551

Thank you for purchasing this product!

HCPro

Roles and Responsibilities of the Peer Review/Quality Committee

Note: The committee responsible for assessing and tracking practitioner performance is often called the "medical staff quality committee" or the "medical staff peer review committee." Throughout this text, the committee will be referred to as the "medical staff peer review committee."

When most people think of peer review, they envision a group of practitioners sitting around a table looking at charts. In reality, peer review has evolved into a much more complex process. A more contemporary definition of peer review is the evaluation of a practitioner's performance for all defined competency areas, using multiple data sources.

This modern definition of peer review implies that clinical knowledge is not the only practitioner competency. Rather, practitioners are now evaluated based on six competency areas that The Joint Commission and the Accreditation Council for Graduate Medical Education have identified. This new definition also implies that case review is only part of peer review. Case review is an important part of peer review, but there are other tools, such as rate and rule indicators, that provide a more fair and balanced view of practitioner performance.

Also consider the definition of a peer, which has also changed over time. In the past, a peer was a practitioner in the same specialty, *old* because practitioners believe that only another practitioner in the same specialty can adequately evaluate their care. In reality, it takes a more flexible definition of a peer to make peer review effective. Just because a neurosurgeon performs a procedure does not mean that a neurosurgeon must review a case in its entirety. For example, if the issue is one of whether the neurosurgeon used the correct size shunt for the ventricle to reduce hydrocephalus, then one would presume (and would be correct) that another neurosurgeon should review the case. However, if the issue is how the neurosurgeon managed postoperative anticoagulation or preoperative cardiac clearance, certainly other physicians could act as peers, because they would have the content expertise to evaluate those issues.

The Joint Commission has also redefined peer review over the last few years by introducing the following terms:

- **Ongoing professional practice evaluation (OPPE):** The routine process of monitoring the current clinical competency of medical staff members. It is what medical staffs traditionally think of as "peer review."

- **Focused professional practice evaluation (FPPE):** The Joint Commission uses the same term to describe two different types of peer review. One type of FPPE addresses concerns raised about a practitioner's performance during OPPE. The second type of FPPE applies to new medical staff members or those requesting new privileges. For a focused period of time, medical staffs must evaluate practitioners' performance to ensure that they made an informed decision when granting or denying a practitioner privileges.

- **General competencies:** The general competencies provide the framework for measuring and evaluating practitioners. The competencies are:

  - *Patient care*

  - *Medical knowledge*

  - *Practice-based learning and improvement*

  - *Interpersonal and communication skills*

  - *Professionalism*

  - *Systems-based practice*

When it comes to conducting effective peer review through ongoing and focused professional evaluation for current medical staff members, there are three components. They are:

- **Systematic measurement:** The peer review committee needs a process to obtain performance data regularly and consistently.

- **Systematic evaluation:** The peer review committee must ensure that policies and procedures allow the committee to evaluate practitioner performance using good data. The data must allow the committee to routinely identify outlying performance—both good and bad.

- **Systematic follow-through:** The peer review committee must establish policies defining who will follow up with a practitioner whose performance raises a red flag and when this follow-up will occur. Policies should also detail at what point the committee will take further action when a performance concern is raised.

How Will Modern Definitions of Peer Review Affect Your Peer Review Program?

Many organizations are already conducting FPPE and OPPE, so the modern definition of peer review should not affect them. However, it will affect organizations that traditionally relied on chart review, because The Joint Commission requires that organizations go beyond simply evaluating the same data more often. Organizations must go beyond case review to look at aggregate data (i.e., rate and rule indicators, which we will discuss later in this chapter) and evaluate physicians using all six competencies. Medical staffs must also establish policies that identify when it is necessary for medical staff leaders to conduct follow-up on FPPE results (i.e., how many deviations will trigger the peer review committee to dig deeper?).

What Are the Goals of a Great Peer Review Program?

The goals of any peer review committee should include the following:

- To create a nonpunitive culture that results in performance improvement. This does not mean that the committee doesn't take action when necessary, but it follows a process that allows practitioners an opportunity to improve before taking action.

- To create effective and efficient committee structures and processes. The committee shouldn't waste practitioners' time by having too many subcommittees or meetings that run long because it is reviewing cases that don't need to be reviewed.

- To establish valid and accurate practitioner performance measures. If the peer review committee is going to measure practitioner performance, it must ensure that the selected measures accurately measure practitioner performance at the aggregate and individual levels.

- To provide practitioners with timely and useful feedback. If practitioners are going to improve, they need to understand their own performance data and receive it in time to do something about it.

- To create well-designed and collegial performance improvement strategies to ensure that when a practitioner's performance is lacking, he or she views it as an opportunity for improvement.

- To collect reliable data for ongoing evaluation and reappointment. Yes, peer review committees in hospitals that are Joint Commission–accredited must meet The Joint Commission's standards for reappointment, but if the peer review committee achieves the other five goals, compliant reappointment processes will occur naturally.

The Power of the Pyramid

The performance pyramid describes how medical staffs can achieve a nonpunitive culture. By spending more time on the lower, bigger layers of the pyramid, medical staffs will rarely have to spend time on the top layers. Let's review each layer of the pyramid that appears in Figure 1.1.

Figure 1.1

THE PHYSICIAN PERFORMANCE PYRAMID

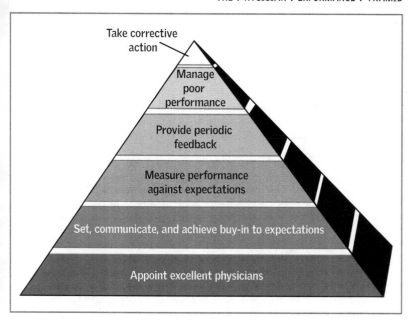

1. **Appoint excellent practitioners.** This layer focuses on the medical staff's credentialing processes to ensure that applicants meet the medical staff's eligibility criteria.

2. **Set, communicate, and achieve buy-in to expectations.** Many organizations make the mistake of measuring practitioner performance without setting performance expectations or defining what areas of practice should be measured and why.

3. **Measure practitioner performance.** Measuring practitioner performance is best done using a clear set of performance expectations and a good rationale for measuring each indicator.

4. **Provide periodic feedback.** Periodic feedback drives a performance improvement culture. Not only is it important for practitioners to see their own performance data, but they should receive both positive and negative feedback. In any performance improvement process, people need to know when they are excelling and not just hear the bad news.

5. **Manage poor performance.** Although medical staff leaders hope that providing practitioners with performance feedback will spur them to self-improve, some practitioners do not understand what they need to do or are somewhat reluctant to do it. They may need additional assistance from key medical staff leaders. Medical staff leaders should partner with these practitioners to help them improve their performance.

6. **Take corrective action.** Unfortunately, some practitioners are unwilling or unable to improve their performance. Taking corrective action, such as suspending privileges, is an option only after the medical staff has provided the practitioner with ample opportunity to improve his or her performance.

How Can the Medical Staff Develop a Nonpunitive Culture?

Creating a nonpunitive culture does not mean looking the other way when practitioners make mistakes. Rather, it is establishing fair and efficient measurement systems to make sure the peer review committee is capturing data that paints an accurate picture of practitioner performance. For example, it's unfair to attribute a C-section to a hospitalist who merely consulted.

The second aspect of creating a nonpunitive culture is to use data evaluation systems that improve physician performance and accountability.

Primary Responsibilities of an Effective Medical Staff Quality Committee

There are three areas that help to drive a great physician performance program. They are:

- Measurement system management

- Evaluation of practitioner performance

- Improvement opportunity accountability

Measurement system management

Let's talk about each one of these in more depth, starting with measurement system management. The peer review committee is responsible for reviewing all indicators, the attribution of those indicators, and the targets that are used to measure practitioner performance at least annually. Typically, peer review committees simply look at a list of indicators and approve them, but the medical staff as a whole needs to be more engaged in the decisions regarding attribution and defining the targets that constitute excellent and acceptable performance.

The medical staff should also be involved in defining and designing the screening tools and referral systems that are used for case review. Department chairs and medical staff members should always be allowed to provide input into the measurement system management process. For example, if a department chair feels that the indicators chosen for a specialty create an inaccurate picture of practitioner performance, he or she should be allowed to present a case to the peer review committee for consideration.

As needed, the peer review committee approves requests for additions or deletions to medical staff indicators, criteria, or targets. Over the course of the year, new ideas come up that weren't discussed or identified previously. These ideas should be vetted through the peer review committee to ensure the best use of the hospital's quality resources.

The peer review committee also designs and/or approves focused studies (FPPE) when necessary to further analyze a practitioner's performance. With the credentials committee, the peer review committee defines the appropriate content for OPPE and practitioner performance feedback reports.

Evaluation of practitioner performance

Evaluating practitioner performance involves two components:

- **Individual case evaluation.** The peer review committee reviews practitioner performance based on individual case review and obtains input from the practitioners as to why certain outcomes occurred. Practitioner input is extremely important, and we will discuss where that comes into the process later in this chapter.

  During individual case evaluation, the peer review committee decides whether the care a practitioner provided was appropriate. The committee also triggers FPPE studies when needed to determine if improvement opportunities exist.

  Although it is not the peer review committee's job to identify potential hospital system or nursing practice improvement opportunities during the course of individual case review, practitioners may identify such issues. These concerns must be passed on to the appropriate leaders to address. The peer review committee needs to hold those leaders accountable to help improve systems in which practitioners treat patients.

- **Evaluation of aggregate data.** The second component of practitioner performance evaluation is the evaluation of aggregate data. There are several steps to evaluating aggregate data. First, the peer review committee must regularly review the medical staff rule and rate indicator data, or it may delegate this task to a subgroup or individual to ensure that it is done properly.

  Second, the peer review committee identifies potential opportunities for individual practitioners to improve. It may determine that an FPPE study is needed because the data has shown that a practitioner has exceeded a rate beyond what is expected.

  Third, the peer review committee should identify the potential for medical staff–wide improvement opportunities. Perhaps the individual practitioner performance data look fine, but the overall medical staff is not performing as well as it could. As a result, the organization must determine how to improve the group's performance.

  Lastly, by evaluating aggregate data, the peer review committee identifies opportunities for the hospital system or the nursing practice to improve. For example, perhaps the lab is not staffed adequately during the hospital's peak hours, therefore delaying test results and, thus, diagnoses.

Improvement opportunity accountability

Although it is not technically the peer review committee's job to direct improvement accountability, it is important that the committee follows through to ensure that the appropriate individuals address issues raised during the evaluation of practitioner performance. When the peer review committee identifies an opportunity for a practitioner to improve his or her performance, it must notify the appropriate medical staff leader (typically the department chair) and ensure that the leader is conducting further evaluation and developing an improvement plan. The committee should make sure that the plan was implemented and report results regarding the practitioner's progress to the medical executive committee.

External Peer Review

Even the best peer review program could use some help, because it can't always perform every aspect of peer review internally. The peer review committee should have a policy that clearly details when external peer review is necessary. There are six common situations that require external peer review. They are:

1. **Lack of internal expertise.** Only one individual on the medical staff can perform a particular procedure or

specializes in a particular area, and the medical staff needs another practitioner to evaluate his or her performance.

2. **Ambiguity.** If differing opinions among committee members render the committee unable to come to a conclusion, an external third party can settle the dispute.

3. **Credibility.** When conflicts of interest arise between members of the peer review committee and the practitioner being reviewed, the peer review committee may need to call in a neutral external party to maintain the credibility of the peer review process and make an appropriate decision.

4. **Legal concerns.** If the peer review committee fears that the physician may be litigious or that corrective action is the next step, the committee may want to cover its bases by enlisting the help of a neutral third party.

5. **Benchmarking.** Having an independent source review practitioner review cases can help peer review committees benchmark their own performance.

6. **Lack of internal resources.** The peer review committee may need to do a large focused evaluation, but it simply doesn't have the time to do so.

Selecting Physician Performance Measures and Targets

Selecting valid and useful practitioner competency measures is extremely important to maintain the credibility of the quality committee. When selecting practitioner quality measures, the peer review committee is trying to answer the following three questions:

1. Who is being measured?

2. What is being measured?

3. How should it be measured?

Who Is Being Measured?

To answer this question, one must understand validity, reliability, and accuracy.

Validity

If a measure is invalid, then the data is not useful. Simply put, if a measure is valid, it measures what it is supposed to measure.

The peer review committee can determine validity using a method called "face validity," which means that on the face of it, an indicator measures what it is intended to measure. For example, physicians are rated based on national core measures, and one of the core measures tracks whether they order particular medications for certain diagnoses. Using face validity, we can say that this measure tells us something about physicians' performance, because only physicians can write orders for those medications. Therefore, it is a valid physician measure.

Reliability

Reliability means that, although the measure is valid and measures what it is intended to measure, it may not always produce a consistent or reliable result. Reliability is the degree to which the performance measure provides consistent or reproducible results. Just because a measure isn't reliable doesn't mean it isn't valid.

Accuracy

Although a measure says something about physician performance and is doing so reasonably consistently, it may not be getting the right physician or the right data at the end of the day. Accuracy is the degree to which the performance measure result is close to the true result.

Physician-relevant measures

To have valid, reliable, and accurate data, measures must be relevant. Physician-relevant measures measure only what physicians have influence over. The peer review committee must select measures for which practitioners are responsible for all or most of the indicator variance. Practitioners should drive the data.

Practitioner attribution

Practitioner attribution is the idea of identifying the practitioner who is responsible for the performance. The peer review committee must have the right information for the right practitioner, and to do so, it needs to have developed reliable and accurate measures. If the peer review committee has valid data that are not attributed appropriately to practitioners, those data will not be useful in the long run. The data must be reasonably assigned to a specific practitioner or a defined group of practitioners who are responsible for the results.

What Is Being Measured?

The first step to answering this question is having a clear understanding of the framework that defines the competency measures the peer review committee is looking for. The following are the six core competencies adopted by The Joint Commission in 2006:

- Patient care

- Medical/clinical knowledge

- Interpersonal and communication skills

- Professionalism

- Systems-based practice

- Practice-based learning and improvement

The six core competencies were initially developed for residency programs through the Accreditation Council for Graduate Medical Education (ACGME). In collaboration with the American Board of Medical Specialties, the ACGME introduced the competencies in 1998. The residency programs have applied the competencies to determine the effectiveness of residency training, and licensing boards are currently applying the competencies to the maintenance of the certification process. Using the six core competencies as a practitioner performance framework is not just a Joint Commission requirement—it is a best practice, and many physician-driven organizations are using the competencies to gauge practitioner performance.

These six competencies go beyond the definition of a good technically talented, knowledgeable practitioner. To provide good-quality care, practitioners are expected to communicate and interact well with staff and patients. They are expected to have a good professional attitude, be responsive, and behave appropriately when they are in an organizational setting. Practitioners must understand that they practice medicine within the context of hospital systems, must follow safety procedures, and must share resources with others.

Finally, practitioners are expected to learn from their experiences and improve.

The peer review committee should select performance indicators using the six core competencies as a guide. To do this well, the committee must:

- Define practitioner competency expectations so it can select the right measures

- Determine which measures currently in use address each of the competency expectations so that the committee can apply them to the correct context

- Decide what additional measures fill in the gaps and add value to the peer review process

Let's use the patient care core competency as an example. According to The Joint Commission, practitioners should provide patient care that is compassionate, appropriate, and effective for the promotion of health, the prevention of illness, the treatment of disease, and care at the end of life. What competencies should the peer review committee expect from this statement? Primarily, it should expect physicians to provide care effectively, use the appropriate procedures or treatments, and do so in a compassionate manner.

How might the peer review committee measure effectiveness, appropriateness, and compassion? To measure the effectiveness of the care a practitioner provides, the committee must measure outcomes. Getting information, such as risk-adjusted mortality data, provides the committee with a measure of effectiveness. To judge whether a practitioner provided appropriate care, the committee might look at indications for procedures or transfusions not meeting criteria. Compassion is about how the practitioner is perceived by those they care for, and this information can come from patient satisfaction surveys and patient complaints and compliments.

How Should It Be Measured?

To answer this question, it is important to understand the following three types of physician competency indicators:

Review indicators are what hospitals traditionally use to identify cases for review. Case review should be restricted to unusual or complex events, with the idea that the peer review committee should be reviewing cases only to answer why something unusual happened in the hands of a good physician. Unfortunately, review indicators, while they get into the details of care, are biased against high-volume physicians, especially when evaluating routine complications.

Rule indicators identify when a practitioner has violated an important policy or procedure. The incident didn't necessarily result in patient harm, but the practitioner should still receive immediate feedback and education so that he or she can self-correct. The committee should send practitioners a letter, typically once a month, to define which policies (if any) they have not complied with and provide them the information (either policy or guidelines) to help them improve. When using rule indicators, it is important to set a target for how many rule violations trigger further intervention by the peer review committee. These letters do not go in the practitioner's file; rather, they are considered educational until the practitioner exceeds a target.

Whereas review indicators ask why an event happened, **rate indicators** ask how frequently something happens. Rate indicators, which require a numerator and denominator, measure performance in areas where mistakes can happen, even in the hands of a good physician. For example, how often do gynecologists nick the bladder during the course of surgery? How often do general surgeons nick the bowel during the course of colon surgery? The question is not whether they happen, but how frequently do they happen? Are they happening more to one physician more than others? Rate indicators are a much more fair approach to physician performance evaluation, because they level the playing field.

Case review indicators

What makes a good case review indicator? The most important thing is to define primary indicators that make the case worthy of review. To be worthy of review, a case should:

- Represent a potential practitioner care issue

- Involve a significant process or outcome

- Not be a volume-based frequency that should be measured by a rate

- Not be solely a policy/clinical practice compliance issue that can be abstracted by a nonphysician reviewer to determine whether care was appropriate, because that could be addressed using a rule indicator

Once the peer review committee has defined a case review indicator, the next step is to define the clinical issues that are included and excluded so that the committee isn't wasting time on unnecessary reviews. Let's use unexpected deaths of medical inpatients as an example of a review indicator with defined inclusion/exclusion criteria.

Inclusion criteria for unexpected deaths might include diagnosis-related groups (DRG) in which the probability of death is low. Exclusion criteria might include deaths in DRGs with high expected death rates (acute myocardial infarction, congestive heart failure). The peer review committee wouldn't automatically have to review every case in high-risk DRGs, assuming there were no practitioner performance issues. Some deaths involving acute myocardial infarction patients might be reviewed because of other issues, such as a missed diagnosis. But the peer review committee can routinely exclude cases in which death is not uncommon and reduce the burden on practitioners to conduct that review.

Other exclusion criteria for death cases might include cases involving palliative care or hospice, because death is imminent. Severe trauma may also be excluded when it is clear that there isn't much the medical staff can do, other than their very best, to save the patient under very difficult circumstances. When a patient presents in the emergency department with cardio pulmonary arrest, practitioners may do their best, but there is often very little that can be done to change the outcome of the care, and thus, such cases would be excluded from review.

By defining clear case review criteria, the peer review committee can:

- Improve case identification by referral sources, because the sources know what the committee is looking for

- Increase inter-rater reliability

- Decrease unnecessary physician reviews by excluding cases that don't need to be reviewed

- Prevent overuse of the case review process

- Increase the medical staff's sense of fairness regarding why cases are selected for review, which helps all physicians feel that they are treated equally

Using rule indicators

Rule measures reduce unneeded physician case reviews and committee discussion, because the committee is sending letters to physicians who violate rules to educate them before they are called before the committee. When using rule indicators, there is no need to collect denominator data; rather, the data are collected through incident reporting systems. Rule indicators rely mostly on event reporting or data abstraction systems that are already in place and are therefore easy to implement.

Rapid feedback equals rapid change in terms of physician performance. We don't have to wait for six months or a year to get an overall picture of practitioner performance, like we would with review or rate indicators. The committee can let physicians know that they need to comply with a policy or procedure issue right away.

Using rate indicators

Most practitioners are familiar with using rates (numerators, dominators, and averages), but the following are some tips for using rates more effectively:

- When using rate indicators, be sure the question being asked has some frequency of occurrence, even for a good physician.

- It is easier to collect numerators and denominators using electronic data. Also, the committee should try to get numerators and denominators from the same source so that it isn't mixing apples and oranges.

- Lastly, use rolling time periods to increase denominator volume. If the committee is looking at time periods that are too short, such as every month or two, there may be little physician volume, and the data bounces all over the place. Consider using a rolling six months, one year, or two years. That way, no matter when the committee looks at the data, it always has six months', one year's, or two years' worth of information. This approach gives the committee higher denominators and makes the data more accurate.

Reducing Bias in Data Interpretation

With regard to aggregate data, some practitioners are concerned about bias. The question is, how do you know what good data look like? Many medical staffs receive reports from the peer review committee that provide data for individual practitioners as well as the medical staff as a whole, but the committee hasn't defined which data require action on the part of medical staff leaders. As a result, department chairs may respond variably from department to department. Departments may even respond differently from one year to the next, because department chairs change, and the new chair might have different ideas about when action is necessary.

These problems can easily be taken care of by taking the time up front to set prospective targets (we will discuss what kind of targets to set later in this chapter). Targets help the peer review committee define what good performance looks like. Comparative data doesn't tell you what good performance looks like; it only compares one practitioner's performance to others' performance. The mean only tells you what the middle is, but the target defines the goal. Targets are a cultural choice; the medical staff chooses targets based on what it believes good performance should look like.

When choosing the number of targets, most medical staffs think, "We just need a target to identify a performance issue and tell us when to respond." But if you are designing your practitioner performance improvement program to give practitioners feedback on their data and to create a performance improvement culture, you want to be able to give them positive feedback and not just respond when a target indicates a problem. If the peer review committee only sets one performance target, it only creates two zones: acceptable and unacceptable performance. This approach focuses on the "bad apples" and assumes everyone else is okay (see Figure 2.1).

Setting two targets, one for excellent performance and one for acceptable performance, results in the following three zones:

1. Excellent performance

2. Acceptable performance

3. Needs follow-up

The peer review committee should recognize practitioners who are performing above the curve, and those physicians are identified

Figure 2.1   HOW MANY TARGETS: EFFECT ON YOUR MEDICAL STAFF CULTURE

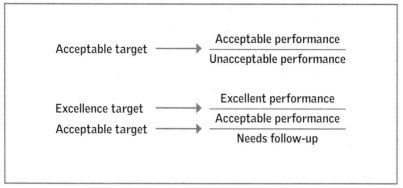

in the first zone (excellent performance). These physicians should know that the organization recognizes and appreciates their performance. The committee wants to send physicians who fall in the middle zone (acceptable performance) the message that they earned a "C" grade. Physicians who fall in this zone are average. The committee wants to stimulate their drive personally and professionally toward self-improvement. Department chairs are not going to talk to physicians in this zone about their performance, but physicians will hopefully seek information about how they can improve on their own.

Practitioners who fall into the third zone require follow-up. The committee shouldn't assume that all practitioners who fall into this zone are performing poorly. Rather, the committee must find out what the data mean and work with practitioners to make any necessary improvements.

Targets for each review indicator are unnecessary, but the committee should set targets for the results of the case review process. For example, when considering the number of cases involving inappropriate care, a target of zero during a one-year period would be considered excellent performance. Most practitioners don't have any cases of inappropriate care, but two would be acceptable in a one-year period for many medical staffs. This indicator says to practitioners that the organization understands and will deal with the individual cases involving inappropriate care, but any more than two cases will trigger the medical staff to conduct a focused study to find out what is going on.

As seen in Figure 2.2, an example of a rule indicator target is the number of blood transfusions not meeting criteria. The

Figure 2.2

EXAMPLES OF INDICATOR TARGETS

Indicator type	Indicator	Target: Excellent	Target: Acceptable
Review indicator	Number of cases with inappropriate care	0 per year	2 per year
Rule indicator	Number of transfusions not meeting criteria	2 per year	6 per year
Rate indicator	Percentile rank for ACEI in CGD	90th percentiles	50th percentile

organization may determine that up to two per year would constitute excellent performance, because even the best practitioners may not always meet criteria for blood use. Acceptable performance might be six per year. The department chair should speak to any practitioner who has more than six instances of inappropriate blood use. The practitioner should have received a letter after each instance that provided education and motivation to improve his or her performance.

As previously stated, targets are a cultural choice. At some hospitals, blood use may be very controlled, and a target of zero to indicate excellent care may be appropriate, because a large percentage of medical staff members never have issues with blood criteria. Acceptable performance may be three or four per year. These are the choices each medical staff makes depending on how the system operates.

Setting targets for rate indicators is a little different than for rule or review indicators. For example, the peer review committee might want to use a percentile ranking to establish targets for using angiotensin-converting enzyme (ACE) inhibitors for congestive heart failure patients. Excellent performance may be in the 90th percentile nationally, and acceptable performance may be in the 50th percentile.

The medical staff might also say that it wants to hold practitioners accountable only for ensuring that the organization as a whole

Figure 2.3

PHYSICIAN FEEDBACK REPORT

Physician Feedback Report

Provider: Anderson, Hugh   **ID:** 38798   **Specialty:** Internal Medicine

Activity

Time Period	Indicator		Volume
1 Yr End 2007 Qtr 4	101	# of Inpatient Admissions	200
1 Yr End 2007 Qtr 4	102	# of Procedures	80
1 Yr End 2007 Qtr 4	103	# of Consults	12

Pt. Care

Time Period	Indicator		Indicator Type	Numerator	Actual	Expected	Index	Acceptable Value	Excellence Value	Score
1 Yr End 2007 Qtr 4	38	Blood component use not meeting appropriateness criteria excluding autologous units	Rule	1	0.02	0.02	0.02	6	2	Green
1 Yr End 2007 Qtr 4	32	# of case reviews deemed care inappropriate	Rule	1	1.5%	0.7%	2.4	2	0	Yellow

Time Period	Indicator		Indicator Type	Volume	Numerator	Results	Acceptable Value	Excellence Value	Score
1 Yr End 2007 Qtr 4	63	Severity adjusted complications index: DRG 89	Rate	41	1	100.0%	1.25	0.85	Green
1 Yr End 2007 Qtr 4	105	Severity-Adjusted Mortality Index: DRG 89	Rate	214	1		1.5	1.0	Red

Medical Knowledge

Time Period	Indicator		Indicator Type	Numerator	Volume	Results	Acceptable Value	Excellence Value	Score
1 Yr End 2007 Qtr 4	104	% required annual CME credits	Rate	50	50	100.0%	95.0%	100.0%	Green
1 Yr End 2007 Qtr 4	106	% HF patients prescribed ACEI at D/C	Rate	175	200	87.5%	85.0%	95.0%	Yellow
1 Yr End 2007 Qtr 4	107	% AMI patients prescribed beta blocker at discharge	Rate	190	200	95.0%	85.0%	95.0%	Green

Practice Based Learning and Improvement

Time Period	Indicator		Indicator Type	Numerator	Volume	Results	Acceptable Value	Excellence Value	Score
1 Yr End 2007 Qtr 4	108	% excellent ratings on feedback report	Rate	130	200	65.0%	50.0%	80.0%	Yellow

Key: Green = Excellence; Yellow = Acceptable; Red = Needs attention

Monday, March 10, 2008

performs at least above average. Perhaps it considers excellent performance to be in the 75th percentile nationally and acceptable performance in the 25th percentile.

Figure 2.3 shows an example of a practitioner performance feedback report that uses defined targets to help practitioners understand where they stand individually and compared to their peers. The green bars indicate excellent performance, the yellow indicates acceptable performance, and the red indicates a need for additional follow-up. This report doesn't leave much room for interpretation; practitioners and department chairs will interpret it the same way and thus can work together to improve performance.

Perception Data

One of the difficult issues peer review committees confront when scoring physician competency is the fact that not all the data can be extracted from the medical record, which was often the case when relying solely on case review to measure practitioner performance. Some of the competencies the medical staff must document and measure can be evaluated only using other people's perception of a practitioner's performance. We call this perception data.

"Other people" include peers, coworkers, supervisors, and patients. All these folks have an opinion of a practitioner's performance and, depending on the questions they are asked, that view may be appropriate. The committee shouldn't ask a nurse or patient whether a surgeon is technically competent, because neither the nurse nor the patient has the education or training to make that determination from a credentialing standpoint. However, the committee can ask patients whether the practitioner communicated with them effectively, or ask nurses whether the practitioner communicates and collaborates well in a team setting.

The core competencies that lend themselves best to using perception data are patient care, interpersonal communication skills, and professionalism. If you look at each core competency statement, you will see that providing good patient care involves compassion, education, and counseling. Interpersonal and communication skills include collegiality and cooperation, while professionalism examines the practitioner's behavior, responsiveness, and sensitivity to diversity.

To measure these competencies, the medical staff must determine what kinds of perception data are available. Every organization collects perception data, whether it realizes it or not. Incident reporting systems that allow nurses to report instances of poor physician behavior are perception data systems. Incident reporting systems are categorized as passive data systems, because the organization has to wait for someone to file a report to identify a problem. In addition to incident reports, complaints and compliments are common passive systems for collecting perception data. The peer review committee can use rule indicators to qualify passive perception data better.

Medical staffs can also collect perception data actively. Active data, such as evaluation forms often used in residency training programs, and surveys, such as patient satisfaction and nursing surveys, use rate indicators to better understand the collected data. Active data provide the sum of many people's views and opinions of a physician's performance in order to create an average score.

Using surveys to collect perception data minimizes personal reporting bias. It isn't one nurse who perceives a practitioner's performance a certain way, but rather many nurses sharing that perception.

In addition to minimizing personal reporting bias, perception data allows normative interpretation to decrease bias. In other words, each physician is compared to everyone else. This is a more powerful data point, as physicians do not like to be outliers. They see how they are perceived compared to their physician colleagues and strive to improve.

Effective Case Review

Case review is only one part of peer review, but it is a very important part, because it deals with serious and complex issues. There are eight key steps to ensure a consistent and fair case review process.

This chapter will walk you through these eight steps and provide you with a framework to develop and/or improve your organization's case review process.

Step One: Identify Cases

The first step of the case review process is to identify cases for review. The peer review committee must document the organization's process for identifying cases for review. There are three common methods for identifying cases. They are:

1. **Automated screening.** Computerized automated screening uses medical billing codes or other information in the

electronic medical record to identify cases for review. This is an efficient approach to screening cases but can identify cases that may not require review. Therefore, the organization should have a second process for screening the cases identified through the automated system.

2. **Manual screening.** Manual screening requires an individual (or individuals) to use an audit tool to look for flags in a random sampling of charts. Alternatively, they may look for red flags in 100% of the charts. Many organizations have moved away from this approach because it is onerous.

3. **Referrals.** A referral system allows people throughout the organization (nurses, case managers, medical records professionals, and risk managers) to send cases through the peer review process. Patients or other practitioners can also refer cases. Using this method, the issues are already somewhat identified but not completely defined until the case goes through the next step of the review process.

Step Two: Screen Cases for Review

The next step of the case review process is to screen cases for review. The goal of this process is to make sure that reviewers are not spending time on unnecessary cases, such as those that do not involve an issue related to practitioner care or cases that are being measured some other way (i.e., a rate or a rule).

The first and most important step at this stage of the process is case elimination. A nurse or medical records professional who is familiar with the criteria for sending a case though the peer review process often screens the cases to eliminate those that don't meet the criteria for review.

Next, the case is assigned to a practitioner reviewer. The prescreeners (i.e., the nurse or medical records professional) assign the case to the appropriate practitioner based on the organization's policies and procedures. For some committees, this might be a particular specialist, but for committees in a multidisciplinary setting, it might be the next practitioner in the rotation.

Third, the committee should not give a practitioner a chart to review without first indicating concerns about the care provided. Without this information, the reviewer may waste a lot of time reviewing aspects of the case other than the ones in question. Provide the reviewer with key questions about what the committee is interested in learning, such as whether particular medication was provided at the appropriate dosage in a timely manner.

Providing the reviewer with pointed questions does not preclude him or her from finding other issues that may arise as he or she reviews the case, but it doesn't obligate the reviewer to go through the entire chart just to find out why the committee decided to send the case through review.

Step Three: Review the Case

Now it's time to review the case. To make the reviewing process consistent, the peer review committee should define in its policy both the location where the review should occur and the time frame for the initial review. It is important to recognize that for a review to be effective, the initial review should take place outside the committee setting. It is no longer considered a good practice to bring charts to a committee meeting and hand them out to the members, who are seeing them for the first time. This practice does not allow for consistent, credible, and thorough reviews.

It is therefore critical to specify in the medical staff's peer review policy where providers can access the charts for review (i.e., in the medical staff services department) or define how the practitioners can access the charts electronically.

The peer review committee must also define how long practitioners have to review the cases they are assigned. Best practice is to allow two weeks to conduct the review.

As part of this process, the peer review committee must ensure that reviewers complete the rating form consistently. To keep the review process moving, reviewers should perform a credible review ahead of time and come to committee meetings prepared to discuss their findings. The reviewer must determine during the initial review whether the case was appropriate or whether further committee discussion is necessary.

Step Four: Discuss the Case at a Committee Meeting

The committee's goal is to determine whether the care a practitioner provided was appropriate. The goal is not to make the final determination but to decide what questions the committee has for the practitioner. It is important to phrase those questions collegially. Instead of asking, "Why didn't you treat the patient with insulin?" ask, "Did you consider using insulin? If so, why did you choose not to use it?"

After gathering input from the practitioner in question, the committee makes a determination regarding the care he or she provided.

Step Five: Seek Input From the Practitioner

The peer review committee's policy must clearly define the methods by which the practitioner should submit his or her input. Many peer review committees have found that asking the practitioners to provide written answers to written questions is the most efficient method and least likely to cause conflict-of-interest issues or delays in the committee process. Occasionally, the practitioner in question will request to appear at a committee meeting to discuss the case, and this may be necessary if the practitioner's written responses are unclear or if the committee has further questions. However, at least for the initial response, written answers should be adequate for the vast majority of cases.

The peer review committee should define the time frame for the practitioner to provide a written response, generally two to three weeks, unless there are unusual circumstances. Practitioners typically don't have a problem meeting that deadline. The committee should not be delayed from resolving a case by a practitioner's lack of response. If the practitioner fails to respond, the committee should make a decision at its next meeting without the practitioner's input.

Step Six: Make a Decision

After the committee finalizes its case ratings and gathers the practitioner's input, it's time to determine the appropriate level of action. Perhaps the practitioner has already acknowledged the issue and is taking steps to improve his or her practice, or perhaps sending the practitioner an educational letter is all that is required. In more serious cases, the department chair may discuss with the practitioner the next steps to improve the practitioner's performance.

The peer review committee may need to refer some cases to the medical executive committee, possibly for corrective action.

Because there are several opportunities for improvement during the peer review process, corrective action is rare.

Step Seven: Communicate Findings

The committee must communicate its final decision to the practitioner. Medical staff members are accustomed to receiving notice when the peer review committee finds care questionable or inappropriate, but peer review committees often find in the practitioner's favor, usually without the practitioner knowing the case was even being discussed. Therefore, the committee should consider sending letters when the practitioners provide appropriate or exemplary care and when the committee determines that the issues identified during case review were not related to the care the practitioner provided.

When rating cases, consider implementing the following categories:

- Care appropriate

- Care questionable/inappropriate

- Care exemplary

- Nonpractitioner issues

Occasionally, the peer review committee will be presented with cases in which the outcomes are adverse, but the care the practitioner provided was not only appropriate but heroic in the face of difficult clinical circumstances. When the committee identifies examples of such exemplary care, it should recognize and commend the practitioner.

Step Eight: Create Improvement Plans

As noted earlier in this chapter, one of the key responsibilities of the peer review committee is to make sure that the department chairs (or whoever is designated in the peer review policy) develops practitioner performance improvement plans and tracks them to ensure they are implemented. It is important that the committee makes clear to the practitioner what he or she needs to do in response to the committee's findings. To make those expectations clear, adopt guidelines for the review process.

Separate Outcomes From Care

Keep in mind that the primary question the reviewer is trying to answer is whether the practitioner's actions and decisions were appropriate, independent of the outcome of care. There may have been a bad outcome, but that doesn't necessarily mean that the practitioner performed poorly. The outcome may have been determined entirely by the patient's burden of disease.

On the other hand, the outcome may have been fine, but the care was not appropriate, and only by chance or care provided by other practitioners did the patient not suffer a poor outco... the committee must look at the appropriateness of care outsi... the outcome. The peer review committee must consider first how to identify cases in which the outcome and care provided are misaligned. It must also seek to understand the provider's rationale for the actions he or she took.

To determine whether the practitioner's care directly influenced the outcome, the committee should consider the following questions:

- Did the practitioner fail to consider an important diagnosis?

- Did the practitioner fail to indicate an important procedure, medical treatment, or test, or was the procedure, treatment, or test not appropriate at the time it was performed?

- Did the practitioner fail to perform an important procedure, medical treatment, consultation, or diagnostic test that should have been performed?

- Was there a problem with the practitioner's procedural technique?

- Was there a delay in diagnosis, evaluation, consultation, intervention, or decision-making that affected the patient's clinical outcome?

estions as a checklist that the

ıtial review of the case. However, best

ions only as a guide.

ıt also understand the practitioner's rationale.

ın the reviewer must ask (considering that all he or

s. on is the chart) is whether there is sufficient documenta. ın to understand the practitioner's rationale for his or her actions or decisions. In other words, relying on the information in the chart, can the reviewer understand the practitioner's rationale? If the answer is yes, the reviewer can move forward. If the chart contains insufficient data, the reviewer must indicate that there are documentation insufficiencies that the practitioner needs to be made aware of. The reviewer must also ask the practitioner questions to fill in those gaps.

Given that the documentation was sufficient or the practitioner provided additional information, the real question that the reviewer is asking is whether the practitioner's rationale made good clinical sense at the time. The reviewer must put him- or herself in the practitioner's shoes. With the time and the information the practitioner had, did his or her actions make good sense? Was the care:

- Consistent with evidence-based medicine or good practice?

- Consistent with medical staff expectations? If there are no clear expectations, does the medical staff need to create some?

If the answer to these questions is "yes," the committee can conclude that the care provided was appropriate.

Keep in mind that the case may involve technical issues that are beyond the reviewer's expertise. If so, it is important for the practitioner reviewer to ask the nurse reviewers, the quality staff, and the committee chair to get input or raise the issue at the next committee meeting.

Underscoring and Overscoring

Underscoring and overscoring are common issues medical staffs must manage when conducting case review. Underscoring, which is the most prevalent and the least addressed, makes it easy to give cases a stamp of approval unless checks and balances exist. To prevent underscoring, the peer review committee can:

1. Discuss every case at the committee meeting. This approach is time-consuming and often counterproductive.

2. Conduct a secondary review of cases in which a practitioner's care is deemed acceptable, but questions remain. The committee chair does not have to review the entire case, but rather just focus on the reviewer's comments and findings on the case review form. The committee chair then determines whether the reviewer's findings

make sense. If so, the committee chair can put such cases on a consent agenda that the committee can later vote on.

If there are concerns that the reviewer didn't answer questions appropriately or the reviewer's rationale was unclear, the chair can reach out to the reviewer prior to the next committee meeting for further explanation. The chair may opt for further discussion at the committee meeting if he or she is uncertain about or disagrees with the reviewer's findings.

Overscoring is a less common issue in a committee setting, because such a setting allows for multiple opinions and viewpoints. The other members' perspectives often balance one committee member's overly harsh view. In addition, in a committee setting, all members can review forms and correspondence and have a focused discussion about the current phase of the case. As a group, the committee refines questions for the practitioner and identifies and manages potential conflicts of interest.

Further, the tendency to overscore is reduced by allowing all committee members to review practitioner input and by restricting practitioners from making a personal appearance before the committee to respond to questions.

Aggregate Data Collection and Evaluation for OPPE

The collection of aggregate data is critical to the process of ongoing professional practice evaluation (OPPE). The key to understanding aggregate data is to first understand normative data.

Normative data are data that compare an individual to others within a defined group. For example, much of the data hospitals get from national core measures are normative data. When making that comparison, it is important to ask:

- What is the group?

- How was the group chosen?

For example, if a hospital chooses to compare practitioner performance to outcomes and mortality data found in state databases, the comparison group is hospitals within that state. If, however, the hospital chooses to use a Medicare database, the group is larger and the data won't include outcomes for patients that do not have Medicare. Thus, if the hospital compares all of its outcomes to databases that include only Medicare patient outcomes, the performance measures may be skewed.

Some hospitals use proprietary databases offered by various software vendors and compare themselves to other organizations that have chosen to also use that vendor. Being aware of this information is important to accurately interpret normative data.

Expression of Normative Data

There are two types of normative data: process measures and outcome measures. Process measures measure processes of care, such as whether a practitioner gives antibiotics to patients in a timely fashion prior to surgery or discontinues them in a timely fashion after surgery; whether a physician ordered the right antibiotic for patients with pneumonia; and how fast patients with pneumonia got the antibiotics once they arrived at the hospital. All these processes are measured in relationship to the middle.

When evaluating normative data, envision that healthcare is a bell-shaped curve. In the middle are the median (middle value) and the mean (average). There is also a distribution on that curve, which is called a standard deviation and refers to how far the data falls on either side of the median and the mean.

However, because healthcare isn't entirely bell-shaped (it is often a skewed distribution), we typically want to look at normative data in terms of how many data points fall on one side of the middle or the other. This method of interpreting normative data results in percentile ranks. The peer review committee is looking at percentile ranks and asking how one practitioner compares with the rest of the group.

A hospital might measure practitioners' compliance with the core measures using percent compliance (i.e., how often did a practitioner prescribe ACE inhibitors for heart failure patients). However, normative data indicates what percentile a practitioner falls into—the 10th, 20th, 55th, etc.—to show how he or she is performing compared to the rest of the group.

Outcome measures are another form of normative data. Outcomes can be affected by multiple factors—not just what the practitioner did, but also the patient's burden of disease and other factors referred to as "adjustments" (for severity of illness in particular). When collecting outcome measures (mortality, length of stay, and complications), adjust the outcomes based on severity.

After the data are adjusted, outcome measures are expressed as the outcome that is being compared (say, 12 deaths) to the expected outcome (10 deaths) to get an index (1.2). An index of 1.0 would mean that the number of expected deaths was equal to the number of actual deaths. An index of more than 1.0 would mean there were more deaths than expected, and an index of less than 1.0 would mean that there were fewer deaths than expected.

Outcome measures can also be reported by variance from what is expected. For example, three deaths were expected and two occurred, so the variance is one. Outcome measures can also be expressed using statistical significance (how a practitioner's data looked in comparison to the normative group).

Hospitals use normative data because it recognizes all levels of performance. Normative data helps the peer review committee find out where the top and the bottom of the performance spectrum is, thus helping to identify not only outliers but also excellent performance.

Normative data is also powerful because standards move as practitioner performance improves and the field of medicine advances. As the field advances, it is important to evaluate not only percentage scores but also percentile scores. For example, if a practitioner had a 65% compliance rate with core measures for ACE inhibitors when the Centers for Medicare & Medicaid Services (CMS) first introduced the indicator, he or she would have been performing well. Now that the measure has been in place for many years, practitioners have to perform at a much higher level to reach the 75th percentile or greater. If a practitioner stayed happy with his or her 65% compliance, the field would have moved past him or her, and that 65% compliance rate is now actually only considered to be in the 50th percentile, as most other practitioners are performing at an 80% compliance rate or higher.

CMS' core measures are one type of normative data, and there are two issues that can affect how practitioners use this data. The first is determining whether the measure is valid. Is it a practitioner-valid measure, meaning, does it measure indicators that practitioners directly affect? Do practitioners drive the performance? For example, many of the core measures come in a bundle, such as pneumonia measures. The pneumonia bundle measures whether the physician selected the correct antibiotic and whether the patient received oxygenation assessment. However, the nurses do the oxygenation assessment. Therefore, the oxygenation assessment is not a valid physician measure. On the other hand, the antibiotic measure is perfectly appropriate and valid, because the physician must choose an antibiotic.

The second issue to consider when using CMS core measures is attribution. How do you decide which practitioner was responsible for the patient care? Depending on what software package the medical staff uses, nurse abstractors may be forced to choose the attending physician by default. Other software packages enable users to override the default, while others allow flexible attribution fields. Therefore, it is important for the medical staff to communicate the name of the attributable practitioner to the nurse abstractors.

For example, in regard to antibiotic selection for pneumonia, the attending physician when the patient is admitted is responsible for administering the initial antibiotics; therefore, that data point should be attributed to the attending physician. The discharging physician, who may or may not be the attending physician, is responsible for providing ACE inhibitors to congestive heart failure patients at discharge and writing the discharge orders. The medical staff peer review committee must discuss with the quality staff and the nurse abstractor to determine what the software's limitations might be and how they can be overcome.

Risk- or Severity-Adjusted Data

Risk- or severity-adjusted data combine administrative and abstracted data and adjust for severity of risk. If medical staffs measured only outcomes without accounting for other factors, such as the patient's age, how he or she arrived at the hospital, and other demographics specific to the patient that might affect the outcome, then practitioner performance data would be skewed. The medical staff applies all this information, from general claims data or a clinically defined specialty database, like the safety data sheet (SDS) database, to determine whether these factors are related to the patient's outcome.

The patient's outcome is considered the independent variable, and the other factors, such as the disease burden, are considered dependent variables. Once those factors are eliminated, what remains is the practitioner's responsibility for an outcome. The hope is that eliminating dependent variables decreases the variance, but it is not a perfect system. Much of the variance is removed, but there is enough left over to help the medical staff define which providers are responsible for the outcomes.

Severity-adjusted data are affected by the following:

- **Volume.** A low volume of patients makes interpreting severity-adjusted data difficult.

- **Documentation of comorbidities.** So much is dependent on documentation and coding, particularly when it comes to claims databases. If practitioners don't document well, they will not get credit for the complications or comorbidities that are necessary to define the severity of illness and that might turn an unexpected death into an expected one.

- **Coding practices.** If codes are not applied appropriately by the coding staff, it can affect severity-adjusted data, because there will be a variance from national standards.

- **Location of outcome.** If the outcome occurs in the emergency department after a patient has been admitted, it is considered a hospital death. If the patient is admitted under observation status initially and death is imminent, the death is not considered an inpatient death and therefore is not included on the inpatient death report. Therefore, understanding and using the systems is important to making sure the data best reflects how practitioners are caring for patients.

Practitioner Attribution

Practitioners want an accurate system for attributing performance data. Attribution is complicated. In addition to the limitations of hospital information systems, hospitals are now taking care of patients in more complex ways. Patients are now typically cared for by a team of practitioners, which makes it difficult to attribute the care to just one practitioner. Case review makes attribution simpler, because it is clear in the chart who did what, but attribution gets muddied when other indicators are used to measure performance.

Process measures aren't so hard, because it is clear which practitioner was responsible for a process. However, outcome measures can be difficult. For example, three or four hospitalists could treat a patient in the course of a two- or three-day period. How should the hospital assign attribution for deaths or outcomes in such situations? To solve this challenge, the peer review committee should engage the rest of the medical staff in defining attribution. Practitioners can help nurse abstractors define more specifically which processes should be attributed to which practitioners. Nurse abstractors shouldn't attribute an outcome to a patient without practitioner input.

Many databases allow users to assign the outcome to the attending physician or the physician performing the principle procedure, which will provide the peer review committee with cleaner, more accurate data.

Group Rates

Because practitioners are working in a team, the peer review committee may need to approach their performance from a group standpoint. A group rate holds all the practitioners in a group accountable for an outcome, because they were all involved, or could have been involved, in the care over time. If the rate is higher than expected, the committee reviews charts to see whether there is an individual in the group causing the problem or whether there is a problem with the group in general. This is the only fair way to deal with groups that are practicing medicine together, since someone has to be accountable for outcomes.

Attribution is still important for practitioners who are not providing care directly. For example, if there is performance variance between two practitioners with the same underlying supervisory capabilities, then the supervision may be lacking, thus accounting for the difference.

Indicator Data Is Zero

Indicator data is sometimes zero. The peer review committee can put zero data on an OPPE or feedback report if the following are true:

- There was an opportunity to have an event. For example, if a practitioner had privileges to perform a particular procedure and he or she performed a few of those procedures, then there was activity specific to that privilege.

- The peer review committee is measuring general medical staff activity or improvements in patient care (timeliness, responsiveness, good behavior, etc.) and the practitioner participated or was involved in patient care.

If either of the two conditions is met, use the indicator as performance data. Zero events for review or rule indicators means that the practitioner had the opportunity to encounter a problem but didn't. The peer review committee should recognize that. For a rate indicator, if the numerator is zero but the denominator is greater than zero, the physician did the procedure and did not have complications. The physician should get credit for that as well.

However, if the practitioner did not have any activity—general or specific to a privilege—the peer review committee can't use it. Zero data should determine whether the indicator is appropriate to the practitioner's specialty. For example, if transfusion criteria are included on a pathologist's performance review form, the medical staff wouldn't ever see inappropriate blood use, because pathologists don't order transfusions. Therefore, transfusion criteria should not be on a pathologist's OPPE report.

Another cause of zero data is inactivity. If the data are privilege specific, but the practitioner hasn't used the privilege in the past six months, does the practitioner really need that privilege? Should that privilege delineation be reevaluated?

The Effect of Imprecise Data

Practitioners often feel that the peer review committee must have precise data to measure performance. But the reality is that precise data isn't necessary. The committee simply needs reasonable data. If the committee waits for precise data, it will never have it, and perfect should never be the enemy of good. Reasonable data is available that shows differences in practitioner performance, and the committee needs to look at the signal-to-noise ratio. For example, is there enough information/variance above the noise of the data to indicate that a practitioner's performance is different from that of the others?

It is often not the data itself, but how the data is used that concerns practitioners. When the committee receives performance data, the first question should not be, "Why is this practitioner bad?" The question should be, "Why are these data different?" When the committee evaluates aggregate data, simply asking why the practitioner is different opens the possibility of exploring that variance and improving care with medical staff buy-in and support. After all, the variance may be attributed to patient or organizational factors, not necessarily practitioner performance.

Lastly, the committee should continuously work to improve data to make it more reliable and indicative of practitioner performance.

FPPE for Performance Concerns

Once the peer review committee has systematically obtained practitioner performance data, it must determine what to do when those data identify a potential concern. This is the concept of focused professional practice evaluation (FPPE). To do FPPE effectively, the peer review committee must have:

- Systematic measurement

- Systematic evaluation

- Systematic follow-through

The peer review committee is especially well positioned to address systematic evaluation and systematic follow-through.

Initiating FPPE

The first question for the committee is when to initiate FPPE based on peer review activities. Keep in mind that ongoing professional practice evaluation (OPPE) is just the start of practitioner performance improvement—it is where the peer review committee begins to identify concerns and issues regarding a practitioner's performance. The committee identifies these concerns either through a single serious or egregious incident or through the practitioner's failure to meet performance targets. Either way, these are the starting points for FPPE.

FPPE is the process of drilling down into an identified concern in order to confirm whether an improvement opportunity exists and determine the cause of the issue. When conducting FPPE, the peer review committee shouldn't assume that there is an improvement opportunity. Rather, it has identified a possible concern, and it is trying to determine whether that concern is legitimate and relates to physician practice. Alternatively, the peer review committee may discover there are other issues regarding the data collection systems themselves, particularly when digging deeper into aggregate data.

Once the peer review committee has determined there is a legitimate concern, it must determine the cause so that it can create an appropriate action plan. Failure to find the root cause of the problem would make it impossible to link FPPE to physician performance.

Reporting Requirements

Remember that OPPE and FPPE are parts of the peer review process. These processes are not considered adverse actions or "investigations." Therefore, a practitioner who is undergoing FPPE or OPPE is not reportable to the National Practitioner Data Bank (NPDB). Some organizations use the term "investigation" loosely in their procedures and bylaws. In the medical staff bylaws, the definition of "investigation" should be restricted to a formal process whereby the medical executive committee (MEC) has been asked to take corrective action against a physician, but it needs further information.

When OPPE data identify a performance concern, the peer review committee must find out more about the potential improvement opportunity by conducting FPPE. Learning more about a performance concern is not an investigation or adverse action, because the practitioner's membership or privileges are not restricted during this process.

Because they are not adverse actions, FPPE reports and evaluations are not reportable to the NPDB. However, the peer review committee may submit OPPE and FPPE information to the MEC and the hospital governing board to keep these groups informed of physician performance monitoring.

Identifying Trends

There are two primary methods of identifying a physician performance trend. One is a run chart (i.e., line diagram), and the other is a control chart, which is a line diagram with statistically determined control limits. The peer review committee can identify a trend using these tools, but it usually takes a reasonable amount of data to do that.

Changes in a physician's performance ratings over time also indicate a trend. For example, think of the three zones on a physician feedback report: excellent, acceptable, and needs follow-up. If a physician's performance fell from the acceptable range performance to the "needs follow-up" zone over a period of months, this is a trend that the peer review committee should monitor.

Connect OPPE to FPPE

If the peer review committee doesn't connect OPPE to FPPE, it is missing what the OPPE process is all about. To connect OPPE and FPPE, the committee must clearly define who is responsible for evaluation and follow-up and what steps the evaluation and follow-up involve. The committee should develop clear policies to answer the following questions:

- What is the follow-up process?

- How does the committee define when follow-up is necessary?

Answering these questions is easy if the peer review committee has defined prospective targets: it follows up whenever a practitioner's performance is outside the targets. Without targets, the committee is relying on individuals and individual department chairs to decide when a practitioner's performance requires follow-up, which creates tremendous variability. Using a variable, subjective approach also requires the department chairs and peer review committee to evaluate every piece of performance data rather than scanning down a list of indicators and finding outliers by looking at the reds (needs follow-up), yellows (acceptable performance), and greens (excellent performance).

Once the peer review committee has settled on targets, deciding when to move forward with FPPE can be done with some degree of flexibility, as long as it is defined in the peer review policy. For example, the committee may determine that every single red score on a practitioner feedback report requires follow-up.

The peer review committee could also decide that it wants to give practitioners a chance to improve and therefore wait for a practitioner to score red twice in a row for the same indicator before following up (keeping in mind that the peer review committee would be reviewing physician performance scorecards about every six months). Although it may seem unwise to wait, the practitioner who scored in the red zone on one report may score in the yellow zone on the next report, which does not require follow-up because the practitioner has self-improved. This approach reduces the burden on department chairs to follow-up with practitioners.

Alternatively, the peer review committee could also require follow-up if a practitioner scored poorly on multiple indicators in the same category. For example, if multiple indicators concerning interpersonal skills and communication were in the red, the peer review committee or department chair should follow up immediately on that overall category. Whatever approach the committee chooses, it should memorialize it in writing so that all department chairs can follow it.

Identifying Trends Using the Practitioner Feedback Scorecard

Figure 5.1 is an example of a practitioner feedback scorecard or physician history report. For the first indicator, this particular practitioner scored in the yellow zone straight across the board, but other indicators went from yellow to red. Both indicate a trend. For the first indicator, the practitioner is trending consistently, and for the indicators that went from yellow to red, a negative trend is developing. If the indicators went from yellow to green, that would indicate a positive trend. You can monitor the categorical information over time using a scorecard like the one depicted in Figure 5.1, or using a line graph.

Figure 5.1

PROVIDER HISTORY REPORT

Provider History Report

Provider: Brown, Jerry   ID: 109   Specialty: Internal Medicine

ID#	Indicator Title	Indicator Type	6 Mo Ending 2008 Qtr 2	6 Mo Ending 2008 Qtr 4	6 Mo Ending 2009 Qtr 2	Acceptable Target	Excellence Target
1	# of Admissions	Activity	36	57	88		
2	# of Consultations	Activity	86	208	197		

Patient Care

ID#	Indicator Title	Indicator Type	6 Mo Ending 2008 Qtr 2	6 Mo Ending 2008 Qtr 4	6 Mo Ending 2009 Qtr 2	Acceptable Target	Excellence Target
5	# of cases deemed care controversial	Rule	2 Yellow	2 Yellow	2 Yellow	4	0
7	# of cases deemed care controversial or inappropriate	Rule			3 Yellow	4	0
8	Blood component use not meeting appropriateness criteria including autologous units	Rule	2 Yellow	3 Yellow	5 Red	4	1

ID#	Indicator Title	Indicator Type	6 Mo Ending 2008 Qtr 2	6 Mo Ending 2008 Qtr 4	6 Mo Ending 2009 Qtr 2	Acceptable Target	Excellence Target
39	Risk adjusted complications index for surgical DRGs	Rate	1.0 Yellow		0.0 Green	1.3	0.9
70	Severity adjusted complications index DRG 89	Rate				1.3	0.9
71	Severity adjusted mortality index DRG 89	Rate	2.1 Red			1.5	1.0

Medical Knowledge

ID#	Indicator Title	Indicator Type	6 Mo Ending 2008 Qtr 2	6 Mo Ending 2008 Qtr 4	6 Mo Ending 2009 Qtr 2	Acceptable Target	Excellence Target
61	% AMI patients prescribed beta blocker at discharge	Rate	100.0% Green	100.0% Green		85.0%	95.0%
65	% HF patients prescribed ACEI at discharge	Rate	77.3% Red	84.4% Red		85.0%	95.0%
72	% required annual CME credits	Rate	0.0% Red			95.0%	100.0%

Practice Based Learning

ID#	Indicator Title	Indicator Type	6 Mo Ending 2008 Qtr 2	6 Mo Ending 2008 Qtr 4	6 Mo Ending 2009 Qtr 2	Acceptable Target	Excellence Target
32	% excellent ratings on physician feedback reports	Rate	100.0% Green	100.0% Green		50.0%	80.0%

FPPE Policy

The peer review committee should create an FPPE policy that makes clear who does what. For example, who decides if additional indicator data are needed? Should it be the committee, or an individual department chair in conjunction with the quality staff or the chief medical officer? Who creates the practitioner performance improvement plan? Should that involve a group, or should it be an individual with group oversight, such as the quality committee? Who ensures that the plan is appropriate? Who tracks the results and determines whether the practitioner performance improvement plan worked?

Before implementing the practitioner performance improvement plan, either the peer review committee or MEC should make sure that the plan is designed to help the practitioner improve or change his or her performance. This responsibility should probably fall to the peer review committee, but it can be delegated to the department chair or MEC for more serious issues.

Maintaining an Accountability System for FPPE

The peer review committee should provide the department chairs who are responsible for designing practitioner performance improvement plans with a deadline. The committee should define when the plan is due and when they will report back to the committee with a progress report.

Line Item Documentation of Findings

The peer review committee must document its findings for all practitioner performance indicators that were marked red on the feedback report. The documentation should include:

- The committee's findings (e.g., the practitioner needs further training in a particular area)

- How the department chair gathered more data to better understand the performance issue

- How the department chairs and committee responded to performance improvement opportunities

The credentials committee may find this documentation useful, because it provides a more accurate picture of a practitioner's performance. Rather than focusing on the red scores, the committee can track a practitioner's efforts to improve.

Ethical and Legal Issues: Discoverability, Conflict of Interest, and Confidentiality

Every peer review committee member must be aware of the ethical and legal issues they may face when carrying out their committee responsibilities and activities. In most states, laws protect peer review activities, but the committee and its members must still take precautions to maintain that protection and make it effective.

Discoverability

Discoverability refers to the possibility that the information the peer review committee members generate through discussion and documentation will be used in court by a plaintiff's attorney in malpractice litigation.

Discoverability protections exist because courts and states have determined that it is important for medical staffs to have open discussions about practitioner performance and, thus, peer review information should be protected. Otherwise, if practitioners fear that their words will be used against them in court, they will not conduct peer review effectively. States and courts have tried to balance the availability of discoverable information to the plaintiff's cause with overall efforts to ensure sure peer review is conducted well. In recent years, peer review protections have eroded, as some states have made peer review information discoverable to the public.

Immunity

Immunity is different from discoverability. Immunity is a source of protection for members of the peer review committee. It cannot protect an individual or hospital from being sued (anybody can be sued for anything). However, it does protect the hospital when a practitioner sues as a result of the peer review committee's actions (e.g., the peer review committee recommended that a practitioner's privileges be suspended or terminated). Unless the practitioner can establish an improper process or poor intent, the court will automatically throw out the suit.

Immunity comes from the Health Care Quality Improvement Act of 1986 (HCQIA), which is composed of two parts. First, physicians were given immunity from damages resulting from lawsuits. Under the act, a suit is dismissed unless it involves willful neglect or a federal issue. Second, HCQIA also established the National Practitioner Data Bank and requires hospitals to report peer review actions, such as privilege terminations and suspensions.

HCQIA defines the constraints the peer review committees must operate within to retain immunity. First, peer review committees must act in the reasonable belief that they are furthering quality patient care. Second, the committee must act only after a reasonable effort to obtain all the facts. Neglecting to obtain a practitioner's input after an adverse outcome, for example, is not a reasonable effort to obtain all the facts. Third, the medical staff must provide physicians with an adequate hearing process. The physician must have an opportunity to provide the committee with information in his or her defense, and if the committee moves to corrective action, then it must provide a hearing. Finally, the peer review committee must act in the reasonable belief that the action was warranted by the facts and the physician was provided due process. In general, as long as the peer review committee follows its policies, and the policies are in accordance with good practices, the committee won't have to worry about immunity.

Confidentiality

Hospitals must keep patient information confidential in accordance with the Health Insurance Portability and Accountability Act of 1996 and the Health Information Technology for Economic and Clinical Health Act of 2010.

Sources of Peer Review Protection

There are several sources of peer review protection, including statutory protection. Every state has a statute describing the protection afforded to peer review documents and findings. Because statutes vary from state to state, it's important for peer review committee members to understand the statute in their respective states.

The second source of statutory protection comes from case law. As courts review cases, the case law begins to change or erode the protections that may have been originally intended. In Kentucky, for example, case law has all but destroyed the peer review discoverability protections, whereas in Florida, Amendment 7 has changed the law so that peer review information is discoverable to the individual patient but it is not admissible in court. Every peer review committee member must know the state's statutes inside and out. For the most part, many states provide strong protections for peer review information.

In addition to statutory and case law protections, institutions have confidentiality policies that protect peer review information. This is where hospitals can become their own worst enemies. Hospitals must design policies that not only keep peer review information safe, but they must also educate physicians, who are oftentimes the largest source of information breaches. The key is to write adequate policies that describe existing protections and practices that support those policies. If peer review practices undermine policies, the hospital will lose its argument in court.

Conflicts of Interest

Every peer review committee must effectively manage conflicts of interest. Medical staff members are ethically obligated to disclose any conflicts of interest they might have so that medical staff committees can make well-informed recommendations.

For example, if a practitioner is presenting information to the medical staff regarding the use of a new pharmaceutical product, he or she is ethically obligated to disclose whether he or she has a relationship with that pharmaceutical company. The medical staff should not dismiss the information that the practitioner provides, but it should review the information with a degree of skepticism knowing that a relationship exists.

With regard to the peer review committee, a committee member must disclose any relationship with the practitioner whose care is under review. Perhaps a peer review committee member participated in the patient's care or has a vested interest in the issues under review. Those relationships affect the committee member's ability to make an unbiased judgment.

There are two types of conflicts of interest: automatic and potential.

- **Automatic conflict:** The medical staff member is involved in the issue or the case either personally or as a first-degree relative or spouse of either the practitioner under review or the patient. The practitioner cannot be involved in any aspect of this review process other than to provide information to the committee as requested. If an automatic conflict exists, the individual with the conflict cannot participate in the committee discussion, case presentation, or vote. He or she can participate either by writing responses to the committee's questions or by appearing before the committee to answer the committee's questions and then be excused. If a member of the committee has an automatic conflict (he or she is the practitioner whose care is in question), he or she would have to follow the same rules as all other members of the medical staff. If the committee members follow a different set of rules, it undermines the integrity of the committee. Although it would be efficient to ask the committee member a few questions while he or she happened to be there, the committee should send him or her a letter, if that's the policy for all other physicians regarding the initial inquiry.

- **Potential conflict:** A conflict may exist depending on the nature of the issues at hand, as well as the practitioner's relationship to the committee and to the individual(s) who provided the care that is under scrutiny. Perhaps a peer review committee member's practice partner or competitor is under review. This doesn't mean that every partner or competitor has a conflict and needs to be excluded. It means that a potential conflict exists and it must be resolved. Potential conflicts can be managed in a variety of ways. First, the committee member must disclose to the committee that he or she is a partner or a competitor of the practitioner under review. Typically, that discussion should occur before the committee meeting so that the committee can decide whether the member can render a fair and reasonably unbiased opinion. The partner or competitor should strive to back up his or her opinions with facts, which lowers the bar in terms of the ability to use partners and competitors. If the committee is aware that a partner or competitor of the practitioner in question is involved in the review process, the partner or competitor can participate. However if the committee determines that there is a substantial potential conflict, it should be treated as an automatic conflict.

Protecting the Peer Review Process

The first step in protecting the peer review process is clearly documenting the scope of peer review activities. Second, the committee must ensure that information requests flow from the committee to the individual reviewer. If groups of individuals review cases together, the committee must designate them to do so.

Committee members sometimes chat about peer review issues outside the committee setting, but this practice is unacceptable unless the committee specifically asks a group of reviewers to meet to discuss a peer review issue. If a designated group meets, it must do so in a nonpublic setting. You can't chat casually in the doctor's lounge about a peer review case.

Committee members should never share documents outside the committee setting. A peer review committee member can't give a peer review file to a nurse or other individuals in the hospital unless they're designated agents of the committee.

To ensure that documents are not inadvertently lost, the committee chair should, at the end of every meeting, collect all copies of peer review materials that were passed out.

Finally, the peer review committee should develop a confidentiality and conflict-of-interest policy that members must read and sign at least annually. Every member of the peer review committee and any other individuals performing reviews need to sign this policy.

In addition to signing the policy annually, the peer review committee chair should remind members of the confidentiality and conflict-of-interest policies at every meeting. That can be done in a couple of ways. The chair can print a copy of the policy for each member to sign, or the confidentiality and conflict-of-interest policies can be placed at the top of the sign-in sheet. The chair can also simply open each meeting with a verbal reminder of the committee's policies and the seriousness of the issues it faces.

To keep peer review protected, the committee must educate all physicians and leaders regarding the peer review committee's policies and practices.